How To Get Cancer?

- The Reverse Psychology Guide to Staying Safe

Title Page

Title: "How To Get Cancer?"

Subtitle: "The Reverse Psychology Guide to a Healthier Life"

Author Name: Ashish Gurram.

Publisher: Ashish Gurram.

#Online   #Public   #OnlineReaders

Copyright Page

Title: "How To Get Cancer?"

Author Name: Ashish Gurram.

Publisher: Ashish Gurram
E-mail ID: ashishchinnu0@gmail.com

Edition: First Edition, 2025.

Credits: Abhishek G, Sriyaa K, Harish P, Teja Richardwyll, Mahitha A, Sai K, Raju G, Bharath B.

Preface

Cancer—just the word sends shivers down spines. But instead of preaching the usual "eat your veggies, exercise, and go to the doctor" advice in a dry, forgettable way, I decided to take a different route: **sarcasm, brutal honesty, and a reality check wrapped in dark humour.**

This book isn't about scaring you; it's about making you **think**—because let's face it, bad habits are easy, and prevention takes effort. Through reverse psychology, exaggerated truths, and a whole lot of sarcasm, my goal is simple: **to make sure you never take your health for granted again.**

If this book makes you laugh, roll your eyes, or—dare I say—change a habit, then mission accomplished. If not, well... at least you can't say no one warned you.

Inspired by few real-life stories in my life. **Relatives**—2 people in the same family, **Son** and then **Mother. Son**, got **diagnosed** by **Colon Cancer** and left the world, while fighting from freaking 10 young valuable years of his life. While he was in last stage of his life, unfortunately his **mother** got **diagnosed** with **Breast Cancer.** While her treatment period, he **lost** his **life** but she didn't give up, still fighting with it, done with surgery, recovering well. I felt, **she survived** from Cancer.

Ya!! Of course, it's their fault—**indiscipline lifestyle choices, bad food habits, of course genetics as well.**

Disclaimer

This book is intended for informational and educational purposes only. It uses reverse psychology to highlight unhealthy habits that increase cancer risk, encouraging readers to make healthier lifestyle choices.

This book is not a guide on how to get cancer (spoiler alert: it's a terrible idea). Instead, it's a sarcastic, brutally honest look at the bad habits that increase the risk—smoking, eating garbage, never moving, and basically treating your body like a dumpster fire. If you're looking for a fun way to scare yourself into making better choices, you've chosen the right book.

This book is intended for **informational and entertainment purposes only**. While it takes a deeply sarcastic and humorous approach to discussing cancer prevention and health, the underlying message is serious: your choices matter.

This is **not** a substitute for professional medical advice, diagnosis, or treatment. If you have concerns about your health, **consult a qualified healthcare professional**—not just Google, not a random wellness influencer, and definitely not this book alone.

The **sarcasm, jokes**, and **exaggerated statements** throughout these pages are meant to make you think, not to offend or trivialize the experiences of those affected by cancer. Cancer is a devastating disease, and my goal is to encourage awareness, prevention, and informed decision-making—just with a little dark humour along the way.

By reading this book, you acknowledge that your health is your responsibility, and no amount of sarcasm (or avoidance) changes that fact. Now, go make some better choices—or at least laugh while considering them.

So, buckle up—this is going to be an eye-opening ride. And who knows? By the end of this book, you might just decide that skipping cancer sounds like a better plan after all.

Dedication Page

To all the warriors fighting cancer and those working
tirelessly for its prevention.

This book is dedicated to **the warriors**—those who have
battled cancer with unshakable courage, facing every
challenge with a resilience that inspires us all. To **the
survivors**, who have stared cancer in the face and refused
to back down, proving that strength is not just about the
body, but the mind and spirit.

To **those we have lost**—the ones who fought bravely but
were taken too soon. Your stories, your laughter, and your
love remain woven into the hearts of those who knew you.
This book carries your memory, reminding us that every
lesson learned, every warning unheeded, and every choice
we make matters.

To **those living in fear of cancer**, unsure of what the future
holds—may this book make you laugh, think, and most
importantly, *act.* Fear is powerless when met with
knowledge, and sometimes the best way to face the
darkness is with a little sarcasm and a whole lot of truth.

And finally, to **everyone reading this**—if this book makes
you reconsider even one bad habit, inspires you to make
healthier choices, or simply gives you a reason to take
your health seriously (even if it's through gritted teeth and
eye rolls), then it has served its purpose.

Acknowledgments

Acknowledge contributors, healthcare professionals, or anyone who inspired the book.

This book would not have been possible without the relentless dedication of **doctors, oncologists, and medical professionals** who spend their lives fighting cancer—not just with treatments, but with knowledge, compassion, and the sheer will to save lives. Your work is the frontline defence against this relentless disease, and we owe you more than words can express.

Gratitude to **health and wellness experts**—the researchers, nutritionists, fitness coaches, and mental health advocates who tirelessly push the message of prevention, often to an audience that would rather binge on bad habits. Your persistence is what keeps people from sleepwalking into disease.

To **wellness podcasters, bloggers, and educators**, who use their platforms to spread life-saving information, often disguised as casual conversations—Gratitude for making science accessible, for cutting through misinformation, and for reminding people that health isn't just a trend, but a necessity.

A special nod to **GenAI** for being the brutally honest, sarcastic, and occasionally ruthless co-conspirator within time period crafting this book. Because if a machine can remind you to stop poisoning yourself, maybe it's time to listen.

And finally, to **you—the reader**. Whether you picked up this book for a laugh, a wake-up call, or a desperate attempt to outwit cancer, you're here. And that means you care, even if just a little. Keep that curiosity alive, make smarter choices, and maybe, just maybe, let this be the book that changes your future.

Why only **Book**?
This book is special to me because it's my first book. Even though I promote book reading, in this digital world being offline and productive has become nearly impossible. So, to encourage offline productivity, I decided to make this content available only in this book. Let's See, if people also follow the rule as well.

Table of Contents

Let's Begin The Book

Chapter 1: What Is Cancer, and Why Would Anyone Want It?

Why any Human wants Cancer or at least even
write Book on it?
Answers: Reverse Psychology!!! My Mate.

Subconsciously, most of the people in the world are trying to get Beautiful aliment called CANCER. Ya!!! Really, Cancer is VIP gate way to infinite Hospital bills, Diagnostic Tests, Doctor Visits, Never-Ending Medical Bills, Sick Energy Levels. Isn't a dream for Life? Yes, right!

We, Humans have a funny way of doing the exact opposite of what we should. Tell someone to drink water, exercise, and eat healthy, and suddenly, they're craving Full Chicken Biryani with Coke. But tell them *exactly* how to destroy their health, and maybe—just maybe—they'll pause for a second and think, " *Wait, do I really want to do that?"* Just that *THOUGHT* can hook Humans at least for a second in this less attention span world.

In layman terms, Cancer is a disease where some of the body's cells grow uncontrollably and spread to other parts of the body. Normally, cells grow, divide, and die in a controlled way, but in cancer, this process goes wrong. The cells keep multiplying when they shouldn't, forming lumps (tumours) or spreading through the blood. It can happen anywhere in the body and can be serious if not treated.

It's a preventable disease. All most all cancers are preventable.

Chapter 2: The Sure-fire Way to Get Cancer—Ignore These Warning Signs

Outline common cancer symptoms people might ignore.

So, you're fully committed to making cancer a part of your life? Fantastic! The best way to speed up the process is to completely ignore all the obvious warning signs your body gives you. After all, who needs early detection when you can just let things spiral out of control? Here's your fool proof guide to ensuring you never catch cancer early—because why make life easy when you can make it *dramatically worse?*

Step 1: Assume Every Symptom Is "Nothing"

That persistent cough? Just allergies.
The weird lump? Probably just a pimple.
Unexplained weight loss? Lucky you! Free diet plan.

Whatever you do, **never** go to the doctor. Those professionals love ruining a perfectly good disease by diagnosing it early, and who wants that? Instead, tell yourself, *"It'll go away on its own,"* and let nature take its course. **Spoiler alert:** it won't.

Step 2: Avoid Routine Check-Ups Like the Plague

You know who gets regular check-ups? People who *don't* want cancer. But since that's not you, go ahead and skip those annoying doctor visits. Pap smears? Mammograms? Colonoscopies? Who needs 'em? Besides, if you don't know something's wrong, it's basically like it's not happening, right? Genius logic!

Step 3: Ignore Unexplained Fatigue—You're Just Lazy

You've been feeling exhausted for weeks, even after getting enough sleep? Clearly, you're just *lazy* or *stressed.* No need to wonder if your body is trying to tell you something serious—just chug another coffee and power through! Ignoring extreme fatigue is a great way to let serious illnesses get nice and comfortable inside your body.

Step 4: Bleeding? Meh, No Big Deal!

Coughing up blood? Probably just a scratch. Bloody stool? Must be something you ate. Unusual bruising? You must've bumped into something.

Blood is the body's way of saying, *"Hey, something's very wrong!"*—but let's pretend it's just being dramatic. Brush it off, and keep living your best *"this is fine"* life.

Step 5: Pain That Won't Go Away? Suck It Up!

Pain exists for a reason—it's like your body's alarm system. But alarms are annoying, so just hit snooze and ignore that nagging discomfort. Whether it's persistent stomach pain, headaches that feel like an earthquake inside your skull, or joint pain that won't quit, just tell yourself, *"Pain is just weakness leaving the body."* Too bad cancer *loves* this kind of weakness.

Step 6: Don't Google Anything—Or Better Yet, Only Google the Wrong Things

If, for some reason, you're feeling concerned, do *not* research reliable sources. Instead, get your medical advice from:

- Random Instagram posts
- Conspiracy theorists who think doctors are part of "Big Pharma"
- That one cousin who swears essential oils cure everything

Whatever you do, avoid actual medical professionals. Their "science" and "facts" will only ruin the fun of ignoring the obvious.

Final Thoughts: A Fool proof Path to Late-Stage Cancer

If you follow these steps, congratulations—you're well on your way to making sure cancer has the time and space to grow undisturbed. Who wants the hassle of early treatment and survival when you can make things *so much harder* later on?

But if, by some wild chance, you actually want to avoid a slow and painful decline, maybe—just maybe—you should start paying attention. Your body isn't sending you these signals for fun. And hey, catching cancer early might just ruin its whole plan.

Your move.

Chapter 3: Top 10 Ways to Destroy Your Health

Smoking & Tobacco – "Puff away! Your lungs will thank you (for nothing)."

Eating Junk Food – "Because who needs vitamins when you can have chemicals?"

Avoiding Exercise – "Sweat is overrated! Sitting is the new fitness trend."

Drinking Too Much Alcohol – "Hydration? No thanks, let's go straight for liver damage!"

Ignoring Sun Protection – "Tan now, regret later!"

Living in Stress – "Because why solve problems when you can worry yourself sick?"

Avoiding Doctor Check-Ups – "If you don't know you have cancer, it doesn't exist, right?"

Surround Yourself with Pollution – "Fresh air is for losers!"

Neglecting Hygiene – "Who needs clean hands and fresh food anyway?"

No Sleep, No Problem – "Sleep is for the weak! Push your body to its limits."

Uhh! Brutal right!! Pretty
Straight Forward!

Chapter 4: Avoiding Fruits and Vegetables: A Delicious Shortcut to Cancer

Emphasize the importance of balanced nutrition while humorously showcasing the consequences of neglecting it.

Who needs vitamins and minerals when you can survive on a steady diet of processed junk, deep-fried delights, and sugar-packed treats? If your goal is to roll out the red carpet for cancer, then congratulations—you're on the right track!

Why Eat Nutrients When You Can Just... Not?

Fruits and vegetables are loaded with boring, unnecessary things like **antioxidants, fibre, and essential vitamins**—you know, the stuff that helps prevent disease and keeps your body functioning. But who wants that? Instead of fuelling your immune system and keeping your cells in check, why not just deprive your body of the nutrients it desperately needs? After all, nothing screams *"I love playing health colour trading"* like skipping anything remotely green.

Step 1: Embrace the Beige Diet

Want to make sure cancer cells have the perfect environment to thrive? Stick to foods that are lifeless, overprocessed, and completely stripped of nutrients. Think white bread, chips, soda, and frozen dinners. The fewer colours on your plate, the better! A bright, colourful diet? That's for people who actually care about their health.

Step 2: Fear Fiber Like It's a Villain

Fiber is known to help clean out toxins and reduce the risk of various cancers, especially in the digestive system. But who has time for that? Instead of keeping your gut happy and healthy, load up on ultra-processed (Soft Drinks), fibre-free meals (Rice) to keep things sluggish. A clogged-up system is a happy system... for disease. Ya!!!!!.....

Step 3: Sugar, Sugar, and More Sugar!

Why let your body regulate insulin and inflammation when you can just pump it full of sugar and let chaos take over? Cancer cells love sugar—they thrive on it. So, if you're really committed to increasing your risk, go ahead and replace those fruits with candy bars, Irony is you can eat Fruit candy bars. Bonus tip, you wash them down with a soda!

Final Thoughts: Your Body, Your Choice (But Maybe Make a Better One?)

Look, no one's saying you have to munch on kale 24/7, but completely avoiding fruits and vegetables is like firing your body's security team and inviting trouble to move in. The good news? You can still turn things around—maybe throw a carrot in there once in a while.

Or don't. After all, *why fight cancer when you can just invite it over for dinner?*

Take it Easy!! It's All real!

Chapter 5: How to Never Exercise and Invite Disease

Explaining the role of physical activity in reducing cancer risks.

Exercise? Pfft. Who has time for that nonsense? Sweating, moving, and using your muscles is completely overrated when you can just sit back, relax, and let your body slowly fall apart. If your dream is to roll out the welcome mat for disease, then congratulations—you're about to master the fine art of doing absolutely nothing for your health!

Step 1: Embrace the Sedentary Lifestyle

Why walk when you can drive? Why stand when you can sit? And why even sit when you can just lie in bed all day? Moving your body is for suckers who actually want energy, strong bones, and a functioning heart. Instead, perfect the **"human statue"** pose—preferably on a couch, surrounded by snacks. Remember, the less you move, the faster your body forgets how to function properly.

Step 2: Treat Your Muscles Like an Ancient Relic

Muscles are overrated, and maintaining them requires effort—yuck. Lifting things? Stretching?

Strength training? No thanks. Let your muscles slowly wither away like a forgotten houseplant. Weak muscles mean poor posture, joint pain, and an increased risk of falling over for no reason. But hey, at least you're consistent towards disease, right?

Step 3: Keep Your Heart on Permanent Vacation

Your heart is a muscle, and like any muscle, it needs exercise to stay strong. But why bother? Let your heart work overtime pumping blood through clogged arteries while you lounge around, binge-watching shows and pretending stairs don't exist. Want an express ticket to heart disease? Skip cardio entirely! Your future self will thank you... in the form of medical bills.

Step 4: Make Sitting a Competitive Sport

They say **"sitting is the new smoking,"** but that sounds like a myth made up by fitness enthusiasts. If you want to truly embrace the **zero-movement lifestyle,** try setting personal records:

- **Longest time spent in one spot without standing.**
- **Most hours scrolling on your phone without moving a single muscle.**
- **Fastest delivery order placed because walking to the kitchen is too much work.**

Keep this up, and you'll be on track for **poor circulation, blood clots, and an increased risk** of every preventable disease known to humankind.

Step 5: Avoid Nature at All Costs

Fresh air? Sunlight? Trees? What is this, a survival show? No thanks! Vitamin D from the sun helps strengthen bones and boost immunity, but who needs that when you have the comforting glow of your screen? Stay indoors, avoid the outdoors like its lava, and make sure your skin never sees the light of day.

Final Thoughts: A Faster Route to an Unhealthy Future

At the end of the day, avoiding exercise is the simplest way to guarantee a future filled with **aches, pains, chronic illnesses, and regret.** Sure, movement might help you live longer, feel better, and avoid countless health issues, but where's the fun in that?

So, keep up the great work of doing absolutely nothing. Your body will definitely let you know how much it appreciates it... eventually.

Hmm!!! Come on Go On!

Chapter 6: Sun Worshippers' Guide to Skin Cancer

Educate on protective measures like sunscreen, hats, and staying in the shade.

Ah, the sun—nature's very own tanning salon, best enjoyed without sunscreen, shade, or common sense. If you've ever dreamed of looking like a well-done tandoori full chicken while also increasing your chances of skin cancer, then congratulations—you're in the right place! Welcome to the **ultimate guide to frying your skin like a pro** and ensuring a future filled with dermatologist visits, suspicious moles, and a potential starring role in a medical textbook.

Step 1: Sunscreen? Never Heard of It.

The easiest way to fast-track your way to skin cancer is to completely ignore sunscreen. Those SPF numbers? They're just suggestions for weaklings who don't want a deep, golden glow (or third-degree burns). Instead, go out under the blazing sun with *nothing* but your fragile skin and a strong belief in bad decisions. Bonus points if you proudly say, *"I never burn, I just tan!"*—right before peeling like an overripe banana.

Step 2: Stay Outside for As Long As Humanly Possible

Doctors recommend limiting sun exposure, which is exactly why you should do the opposite! The best time to soak up the most damaging rays is between **10 AM and 4 PM**, when the sun is at its most brutal. Forget shade, hats, or protective clothing—just stretch out under the scorching sun and let those UV rays work their cancer-causing magic.

Step 3: Tanning Beds—Because the Sun Just Isn't Enough

Can't get outside? No problem! Just hop into a tanning bed, where concentrated UV radiation gives you the express lane to premature aging and melanoma. Scientists say tanning beds are *literally classified as a carcinogen,* but what do they know? Wrinkles and tumours are a small price to pay for that short-term glow, right?

Step 4: Ignore Weird Moles—They're Just "Freckles with Personality"

Noticing a new mole? Is an old one changing colour, getting bigger, or looking a little *too* funky? Pfft, don't be dramatic! Checking your skin regularly and seeing a doctor would only increase your chances of early detection and survival, and where's the fun in that? Instead, just pretend it's fine until you *absolutely can't* ignore it anymore.

Step 5: Laugh in the Face of Sunburns

Sunburn is your body's way of screaming, *"HELP! WE'RE DYING!"*—but don't let that stop you. The redder, the better! Keep telling yourself it'll "turn into a tan," even though each burn **literally increases your risk of skin cancer**. And don't forget the added perks: peeling skin, intense pain, and looking like a human tomato. Worth it!

Step 6: Moisturizer? That's for Quitters.

Sure, the sun dries out your skin, speeds up aging, and makes you look like a leather handbag from the discount bin—but don't let that stop you! Moisturizing and using after-sun care would only slow down the delightful process of looking **50 years older by the time you're 35.** Who needs smooth, healthy skin when you can have deep wrinkles, sunspots, and an increased risk of melanoma?

Final Thoughts: Your Fast Pass to Dermatology Appointments

By following these simple steps, you can guarantee your dermatologist will know you by name—and not in a good way. Skin cancer is the **most preventable** type of cancer, but why avoid it when you can *actively* increase your chances of getting it?

Or... you know... you could just wear sunscreen, stay in the shade, and take care of your skin like a sane person. But hey!!, where's the adventure in that?

Chapter 7: Stress—The Silent Killer's Best Friend

Explaining the link between chronic stress and
weakened immunity.

Offer tips for managing stress while ironically
presenting unhealthy coping mechanisms.

Congratulations! You've chosen one of the most
effective, time-tested ways to ruin your health
without lifting a finger: **chronic stress.** Why let
your body function normally when you can keep
it in a constant state of panic, anxiety, and
exhaustion? If you're looking for a **fast-track
ticket to burnout, heart disease, and an immune
system that gives up on you**, then welcome! Let's
explore how to stress yourself into an early grave.

Step 1: Worry About Everything, All the Time

Bills? Worry about them.
Work? Worry about it.
That thing you said five years ago that no one
remembers? Obsess over it at 2 AM.

The goal here is **never to relax.** If you start to feel
calm, immediately remind yourself of everything
that could go wrong. If there's nothing wrong *right
now*, start worrying about *future* disasters. Your

body thrives on constant tension—so keep those stress hormones (cortisol) pumping!

Step 2: Sleep Is for the Weak

Want to *really* maximize your stress levels? **Destroy your sleep schedule.** Stay up scrolling through your phone, replaying embarrassing moments from childhood, or convincing yourself that minor symptoms mean you have a rare disease. Who needs rest when you can **wake up exhausted and fuel your day with caffeine, anxiety, and regret?**

Step 3: Say Yes to Everything—Burnout or Bust!

You have way too much on your plate? **Perfect!** Say yes to more commitments.
Exhausted from work? **Take on extra projects.** Mentally drained? **Make sure to help everyone else before taking care of yourself.**

Burnout is just a fancy word for **"pushing yourself to the breaking point"**—and breaking points are *character-building*, right? Ignore self-care, avoid boundaries, and remember: **"If you're not suffering, are you even working hard enough?"**

Step 4: Eat Like a Stressed-Out Rat

Balanced meals? No thanks! If you're serious about stress, **fuel your body with caffeine, sugar, and fast food.** Skip breakfast, overeat at midnight, and wash everything down with energy drinks. Malnourishment + high cortisol = the ultimate combo for **heart disease, diabetes, and a digestive system that absolutely hates you.**

Step 5: Exercise? Nah, Just Stay Stressed

People say exercise helps manage stress, but what do they know? Instead of moving your body, **sit for hours, hunched over, scrolling through bad news and fake news.** Let all that tension build up in your neck and shoulders until your body physically *locks up* like an old laptop running too many programs. Pain is just part of the experience! Let's experience it.

Step 6: Keep Your Emotions Bottled Up for Maximum Impact

Feeling overwhelmed? **Bury it deep down.** Never talk about your problems, never ask for help, and absolutely **never** take a break. The best way to maximize stress-related health issues is to **pretend everything is fine** while your blood pressure skyrockets and your heart quietly begs for mercy.

Final Thoughts: The Perfect Way to Self-Destruct

By following these steps, you'll be well on your way to **weakened immunity, high blood pressure, heart disease, and a nervous system that's permanently stuck in panic mode.** Stress won't just ruin your day—it'll slowly ruin your life.

But hey, you could also try **sleeping, setting boundaries, eating real food, and maybe... chilling out once in a while?** Nah, that would make too much sense.

Chapter 8: A World Without Check-Ups: The Ultimate Gamble

Highlight the importance of regular health screenings and preventive measures.

Who needs doctors when you have *luck*? Why waste time on routine check-ups when you can just **wait until something is seriously wrong**? If the thrill of gambling excites you, then skipping medical exams is the ultimate high-stakes bet—because what's more exhilarating than **not knowing if a disease is silently wrecking you from the inside?**

Let's explore how to turn your health into a game of Online Betting—no doctors, no tests, just blind optimism and a whole lot of denial.

Step 1: If You Can't See It, It's Not Real

The first rule of skipping check-ups? **If you don't know about a problem, it doesn't exist.**
That weird lump? Ignore it.
Frequent headaches? Probably just stress.
Unexplained and Unplanned weight loss? A *free diet plan*!

Whatever you do, **never investigate symptoms.**
The less you know, the more exciting life
becomes—because who doesn't love a surprise
stage-four diagnosis?

Step 2: Trust Your "Self-Diagnosis" Over Medical Science

Doctors go through years of medical school, but
you? You have **Google**. Why waste time with an
actual expert when you can:

- Diagnose yourself using WebMD's
  "random symptom generator"
- Rely on that one *Facebook friend* who
  swears garlic cures everything
- Assume you're fine because "it went away
  on its own" (for now)

Medical professionals might catch problems *early*
when they're actually treatable, but that would be
way too responsible, wouldn't it?

Step 3: Avoid Preventative Tests—They're Just Trying to Ruin Your Fun

Pap smears, mammograms, blood tests, and
colonoscopies? Pfft. Those are just fancy ways for
doctors to **discover problems before they become
life-threatening**—and where's the adventure in
that? Instead, play the waiting game and let

diseases get a solid head start before *maybe* doing something about them.

Step 4: Assume You're Invincible (Until You're Not)

The best excuse for skipping check-ups? **"I feel fine!"**
Because obviously, if something were wrong, your body would send you a **big, flashing neon sign, right?** *Wrong.* Many serious illnesses—like cancer, diabetes, and high blood pressure—**show zero symptoms until they've already done major damage.**

But hey, why worry about *prevention* when you can enjoy the thrill of an unexpected medical crisis?

Step 5: Medical Bills? Just Wait Until They're Even Higher!

Afraid of doctor visits costing too much? Great! **Ignoring your health now guarantees you'll pay way more later.** A simple check-up might cost a little, but skipping it ensures you'll eventually rack up **astronomical hospital bills, expensive emergency treatments, and—if you're lucky—a lifetime supply of prescription meds.**

If your goal is **financial ruin through preventable diseases**, then keep doing what you're doing!

Final Thoughts: Health Is Overrated Anyway

By following this simple guide, you can successfully turn your **own well-being into an unpredictable, high-stakes gamble.** Will you be fine? Will you drop dead at any moment? **Who knows!** That's the fun part.

Or, you know, you could **just go for regular check-ups, catch problems early, and maybe not die unnecessarily.** But hey—*where's the suspense in that?*

Chapter 9: The Role of Genetics—Blame Your Parents!

Explaining hereditary cancer risks in simple terms.

Encourage genetic counselling and healthy habits to mitigate risks.

Ah, genetics—the ultimate excuse for everything. Got a slow metabolism? **Blame your parents.** Hairline retreating faster than your will to exercise? **Genetics, obviously.** Higher risk of cancer, diabetes, or heart disease? **Totally not your fault!**

Why bother with healthy habits when you can just shrug and say, *"It runs in the family"*? After all, what's the point of trying when your DNA has already decided your fate?

The Inheritance You Didn't Ask For

You probably hoped for **money, good looks, or at least a decent sense of humour** from your parents. Instead, they handed down a **deluxe package of genetic risks—Like debt, twisted looks, or tumours....** Complete with an increased chance of various diseases and some bonus quirks like near-sightedness or an inability to roll your tongue.

And the best part? **There's no returns or exchanges!** Whatever genetic mess you got, you're stuck with it. Thanks, Mom and Dad!

Why Take Responsibility When You Can Just Give Up?

Science says lifestyle choices can *override* many genetic risks, but why listen to that nonsense? Instead of eating healthy, exercising, or getting regular check-ups, just lean into **fatalism.** If heart disease or cancer runs in your family, **embrace it!** Order that Tawa Bonda with Extra Butter, avoid all physical activity, and let destiny do its thing.

"It's in My Genes" – The Perfect Excuse for Everything

- *Doctor:* You should exercise to lower your risk of heart disease.
    - *You:* "Nah, heart attacks run in my family. Can't fight genetics!"
- *Doctor:* Maybe cut back on smoking—it increases your risk of lung cancer.
    - *You:* "My grandpa smoked his whole life and lived to 90! I'll take my chances."
- *Doctor:* Your diet might be causing your high blood sugar.
    - *You:* "Nope, it's just my genes. Pass the chips, *Doc.*"

Why put in effort when you can **conveniently blame your ancestors for every bad habit?**

The Harsh Reality (That You'll Ignore Anyway)

Yes, genetics play a role in disease. No, they are **not a death sentence.** But acknowledging that means **taking action**, and that sounds exhausting. So instead, keep pretending that your family tree is the sole reason you never get off the couch.

Because hey—if you're going to blame your parents for something, might as well make it *everything.*

Wait!!
Wait!!
Wait For More!

Chapter 10: Turning the Tables—How to Actually Avoid Cancer

Breaking the reverse psychology niche.

Provide practical, actionable advice for a healthy lifestyle.

Wait... you actually *don't* want cancer? What a shocker! Here I was, assuming you'd love the thrill of expensive treatments, endless hospital visits, and a body that betrays you in the worst way possible. But fine, since you insist on ruining cancer's plans, let's talk about so called "How To *not* get Cancer!".

Alright, enough with the jokes. You've stuck around, laughed (hopefully), and maybe even thought, *"Wait... am I actually doing some of these things?"* That's the point.

The good news? **A lot of cancer is preventable.** The bad news? **That requires effort.** (Ugh, I know.)

But don't worry, I'll make this easy for you. Just do the *exact opposite* of what we've covered so far, and you *might* just make it out alive. If you missed it, reread the book.

Step 1: Stop Treating Your Body Like a Dumpster

If your daily diet consists of fried mystery meat, sugar in solid and liquid form, and something vaguely resembling bread, congratulations—you're playing straight into cancer's hands! Cancer *loves* inflammation, processed junk, and a total lack of nutrients.

Want to fight back? Annoy it with:

- **Fruits and vegetables** (Yes, the green stuff you avoid.)
- **Real food** (If it lasts 6 months on a shelf, your body probably hates it.)
- **Less sugar** (I know!!! I know—how will you function without your sugar addiction? Figure it out.)

Step 2: Move Your Body (Yes, You Have To)

Sitting all day is basically an open invitation for disease. If your idea of exercise is walking to the fridge, we have a problem. Cancer *thrives* when you stay as still as possible—so ruin its plans by **moving.**

You don't have to become an elite athlete—just:

- Walk like a person who *wants* to be alive.

- Stretch so you don't turn into a stiff, aching mess.
- Do literally *any* form of exercise that gets your blood circulating.

Step 3: Sunscreen. Use It. No, Seriously.

If you think sunscreen is just for beach days, congratulations—you've just given skin cancer a head start. Those UV rays don't care whether you're sunbathing or just existing outside for five minutes.

So, either:

- Wear sunscreen like an adult who values their skin, **or**
- Age like a dried-out leather couch while increasing your cancer risk.

Your call.

Step 4: Maybe See a Doctor Before You're Dying?

Ground-breaking idea: **go to the doctor before something is *obviously* wrong.**
Regular check-ups can catch cancer early, but sure, let's all just *wait* until we're coughing up blood to take things seriously.

If you actually want to stay alive:

- **Get screened.** (They're not doing it for fun.)
- **Pay attention to your body.** (If something feels *off*, it probably is.)
- **Stop treating check-ups like an optional subscription service.**

Step 5: Cut the Stress Before It Cuts You

Chronic stress isn't just bad for your mood—it's like throwing a party for disease. If your blood pressure spikes every time you open your inbox, congratulations, you're already halfway to ruining your health.

Try this instead:

- **Sleep.** (No, 4 hours is *not* enough. Minimum 6 hours, Maximum 8 hours.)
- **Breathe.** (Holding in stress until you implode is *not* a personality trait.)
- **Say 'no' to things that drain you.** (You're allowed. I promise.)

Step 6: Maybe Stop Poisoning Yourself?

Smoking? Drinking like you're in a club house? Congratulations, you're directly **funding** cancer's plans. It's like giving your worst enemy a winning lottery ticket.

- Smoking? **Just stop.** (No, "cutting back" isn't the same thing.)
- Drinking? **Moderation or Just stop, or enjoy your liver's slow demise.**
- Vaping? **Not "better"—just a different way to wreck yourself**

Cancer is serious. It's not a joke. But learning **how to prevent it** doesn't have to be boring or terrifying. So, let's get real.

Extra Exact Real Information....

1. Quit Smoking & Tobacco – The #1 Cancer Gift Box

- If you smoke, **quit now.** There's no "safe amount."
- Second hand smoke? Just as bad. **Don't be around smokers.**
- Need help quitting? **Use nicotine replacement therapy (NRT) or seek professional support.**

2. Eat Like You Care About Your Body

- **More plants, no processed foods.**
- Limit **red meat & processed meats** (Mutton, Beef, Non-Veg Snacks).
- NO to **refined sugar & alcohol.**

- Instead, fill your plate with:
    - **Leafy greens** (spinach, curry leaves and many)
    - **Colourful fruits** (bananas, berries, oranges and many)
    - **Nuts & seeds** (almonds, flaxseeds, pumpkin seeds and many)
    - **Whole grains and millets** (brown rice, Ragi, Jowar, more..)

3. Move Your Body!

- **150 minutes** of moderate exercise per week = 30 mins, 5 days a week.
- Even small changes matter: **Take the stairs, walk instead of drive, stretch often.**
- Strength training boosts immunity—**lift those weights!**

4. Protect Your Skin

- Use **sunscreen (SPF 30+)** daily.
- Avoid **tanning beds** (they're cancer machines).
- Wear **hats, sunglasses, and cover skin in peak sun hours (10 AM - 4 PM).**

5. Get Your Check-Ups!

- **Early detection** = Higher survival rates.
- Women: **Mammograms & Pap smears.**
- Men: **Prostate exams.**

- Colonoscopies: **After 45 (earlier if family history exists).**
- Skin exams: **Check moles, see a dermatologist yearly.**

6. Manage Stress Like a Boss

- **Chronic stress weakens immunity.**
- Meditate, do yoga, **breathe deeply.**
- Set boundaries: **Study and Mobile or Work and Mobile is not only The Life.**
- Sleep 7–9 hours per night.

7. Your Environment Matters

Avoid exposure to **pesticides, industrial chemicals, air pollution.**

- Drink **clean, filtered water.**
- Store food in **glass or steel or copper, not plastic (especially in microwaves)**

Final Thoughts: It's Literally Up to You

Want to avoid cancer? Then stop *acting* like you want it. It's not rocket science nor cracking bloody entry level job—your body can only take soo much abuse before it gives up on you.

But hey, if you *enjoy* playing a slow game of self-destruction, by all means—keep doing what you're doing. Just don't act surprised when your body

finally calls it quits.
Finally, it's up to you!!..

Think, Decide, Action

Action is important. My Mate.

The typical Indian diet may be praised for its health benefits, but let's be real—it's not a one-size-fits-all solution. Customize your meals to match your body's actual needs, aim for balance, and most importantly, enjoy life without guilt or regret.

Lifestyle Matters. Environment Matters. Genetics Matter.

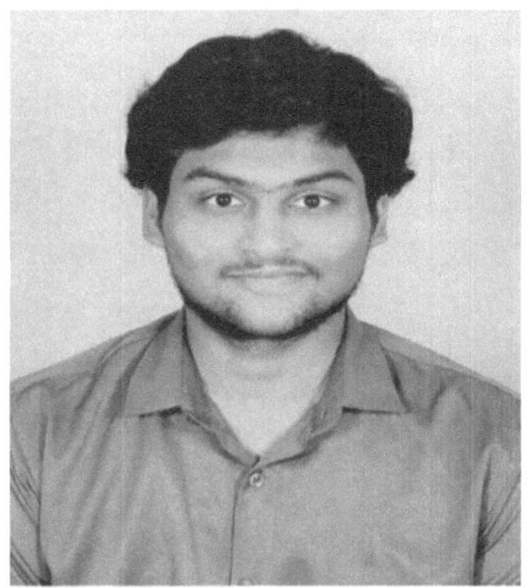

Name: Ashish Gurram
Age: 22 (2025).
Occupation: Entrepreneur.

I, Ashish Gurram, or Gurram Ashish—both names mean the same. Born in what was then Mandal, now a district called Siddipet, Telangana. Raised in another part of the city called Secunderabad, Telangana, because my parents settled here for work purposes.

My childhood was quite the adventure: notorious, funny, known as the naughty kid (Tarzan, Chinpin) of Street 6, Goutham Nagar. At school, I was a pretty average student but still loved by many teachers. I had decent behaviour, was a well-mannered kid, and all the good adjectives fit me when I was at school.

After completing my diploma, I took a 1-year break
due to uncertainties in my life and the world
(COVID). Then, I decided to join engineering
(obviously). I didn't want to waste time traveling to
college, so I picked an engineering college that was
very close to my house in 2021. I'm a pretty average
student here as well, and I'm maintaining it. Proud of
me. But I'm always looking for ways to level up in
life.

After December 2023, I embarked on my fitness
journey. I transformed from 82kg to 64kg (2025),
staying healthy and maintaining it. Now, in 2025,
while writing my 4-1 exams, I decided to start my
wealth journey. So, I began with the basics, from this
book.

I aspire to achieve more in life. Be a part of my
journey in aspects like a friend, family, relative, client,
customer, investor, mentor, boss, employee, or just a
random person. Come, explore, and be part of the
successful journey of an aspiring entrepreneur's life.

#takeapart #entreprenearlifejourney #MAGA
#MakeAshishGreatAgain #behealthy #bewealthy
#wanttobewealthy

The End for **Now.**

-See You Soon

Your Obediently

Ashish Gurram

Scan me and #Feedback

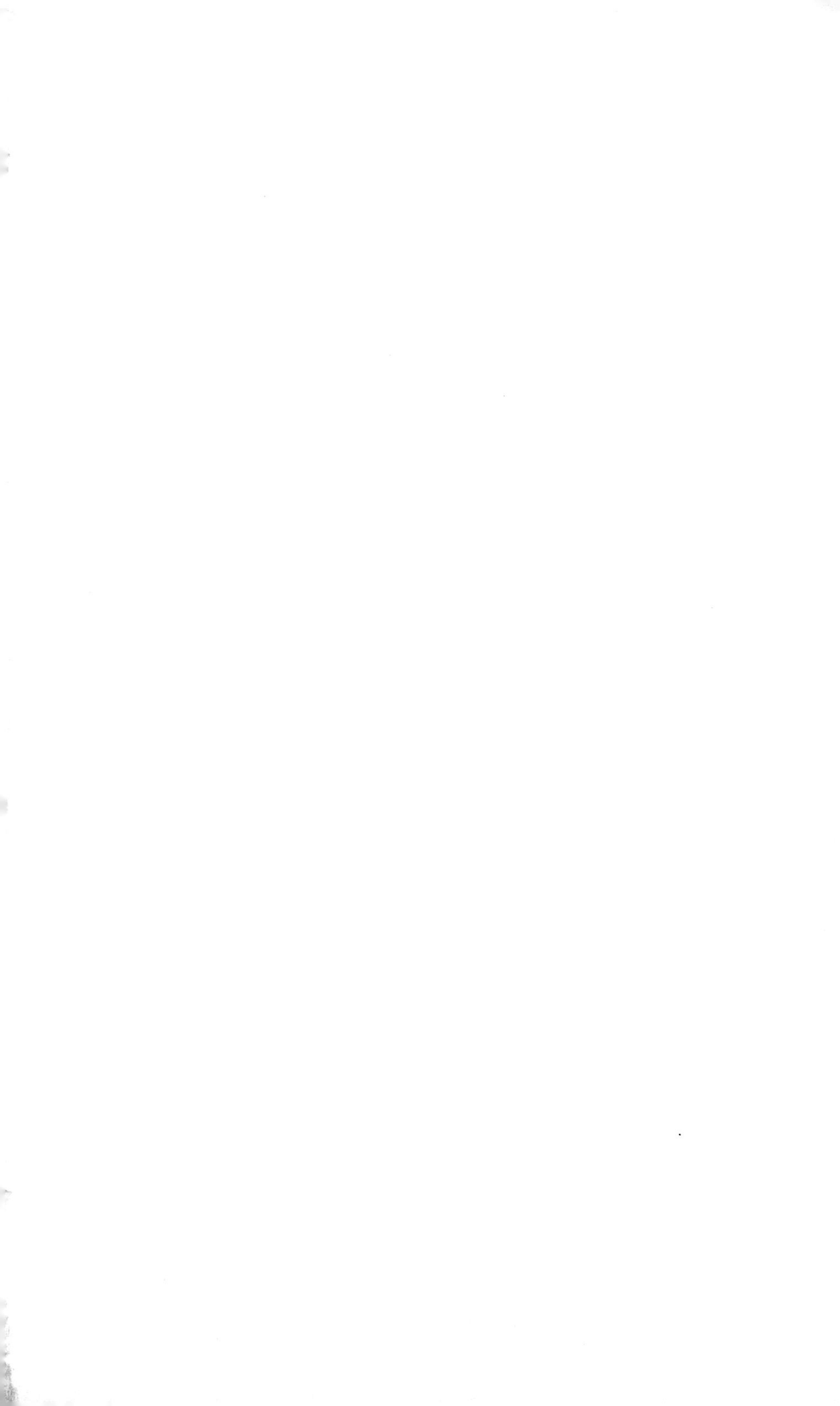

www.ingramcontent.com/pod-product-compliance
Lightning Source LLC
Chambersburg PA
CBHW020513160726
47991CB00007B/2933